Unlocking Your Potential

Self-Care for Teens with ADHD

By

Micheal U. George

<u>Table Of Contents</u>

Chapter 1: Understanding ADHD: An Overview for Teens

What is ADHD

ADHD stands for Attention-Deficit/Hyperactivity Disorder. It is a neurodevelopmental disorder that affects both children and adults. ADHD is characterized by persistent patterns of inattention, impulsivity, and/or hyperactivity that interfere with daily functioning and development.

The core symptoms of ADHD include:

Inattention: Difficulty paying attention, staying focused, and completing tasks. Individuals with ADHD may have trouble organizing and prioritizing tasks, following instructions, and maintaining attention to details.

Impulsivity: Acting without thinking, difficulty waiting their turn, interrupting others, and making impulsive decisions without considering the consequences.

Hyperactivity: Excessive motor activity, such as restlessness, fidgeting, and difficulty staying still or engaging in quiet activities.

There are three main subtypes of ADHD:

- Predominantly Inattentive Presentation: Individuals primarily exhibit symptoms of inattention without significant hyperactivity or impulsivity.

- Predominantly Hyperactive-Impulsive Presentation: Individuals primarily exhibit symptoms of hyperactivity and

> impulsivity without significant inattention.

- Combined Presentation: Individuals exhibit symptoms of both inattention and hyperactivity/impulsivity.

ADHD can have a significant impact on various aspects of an individual's life, including academic performance, work performance, relationships, and self-esteem. However, with proper diagnosis, understanding, and management, individuals with ADHD can lead fulfilling and successful lives. Treatment options may include medication, behavioral therapy, psychoeducation, and support from mental health professionals.

How It Affects Teens

ADHD (Attention Deficit Hyperactivity Disorder) can have a significant impact on teenagers in various aspects of their lives. Here are some ways ADHD may affect teens:

Academic performance: Teens with ADHD may struggle with academic performance due to difficulties with attention, organization, and time management. They may have trouble focusing in class, staying on task, and completing assignments on time, which can result in lower grades and increased academic stress.

- Social interactions: Teens with ADHD may face challenges in social interactions. They may struggle with impulse control, interrupting others, and difficulty following social cues, which can lead to difficulties in forming and maintaining friendships. They may also struggle with managing their emotions, leading to impulsive or erratic behaviors that can impact their relationships with peers and authority figures.

- Emotional well-being: Teens with ADHD may experience emotional dysregulation, mood swings, and impulsivity. They may struggle with managing frustration, anger, and impulsiveness, which can lead to conflicts with family members, friends, and teachers. The emotional and behavioral challenges associated with ADHD can also lead to increased stress, anxiety, and low self-esteem.

- Executive functioning skills: ADHD can impact a teenager's executive functioning skills, which include abilities such as planning, organizing, initiating tasks, and self-regulation. Teens with ADHD may have difficulty initiating and completing tasks, managing their time effectively, and staying organized, which can impact their ability to independently manage their responsibilities and daily routines.

- Risk-taking behaviors: Teens with ADHD may engage in risky behaviors such as impulsive decision-making, substance abuse, and reckless driving. These behaviors may be due to difficulties with impulse control and poor judgment, which can put them at higher risk for accidents, injuries, and negative consequences.

- Self-esteem and self-concept: ADHD can impact a teenager's self-esteem and self-concept. They may struggle with feelings of inadequacy, frustration, and low self-worth due to challenges they face in various areas of their life, including academics, social interactions, and emotional regulation.

It's important to note that the symptoms and severity of ADHD can vary widely among individuals, and not all teens with ADHD will experience the same challenges. With appropriate support, such as medication, therapy, and accommodations at school, many teenagers with ADHD are able to manage their symptoms and lead successful, fulfilling lives. If you suspect that your teenager may have ADHD, it's important to seek a professional evaluation and develop an individualized treatment plan to support their specific needs.

Common misconceptions about ADHD

Attention deficit hyperactivity disorder (ADHD) is a neurodevelopmental disorder that affects both children and adults. It is characterized by symptoms such as difficulty paying attention, impulsivity, and hyperactivity. Despite being a well-researched condition, there are several common misconceptions about ADHD that often lead to misunderstanding and stigma. In this article, we will explore some of these misconceptions and shed light on the facts.

Misconception 1: ADHD is not a real disorder, and it's just an excuse for poor behavior.

One of the most pervasive misconceptions about ADHD is that it is not a real disorder and is simply an excuse for poor behavior or lack of discipline. However, this is far from the truth. ADHD is a recognized neurodevelopmental disorder that has been extensively studied and documented by medical and psychological professionals. Research has shown that ADHD is caused by a combination of genetic, environmental, and neurological factors that affect the brain's ability to regulate attention, impulse control, and behavior. People with ADHD have different brain chemistry and brain activity compared to those without ADHD, which can significantly impact their ability to focus, control impulses, and manage behavior.

Misconception 2: ADHD only affects children.

Another common misconception about ADHD is that it only affects children. While ADHD is often diagnosed in childhood, it can persist into adulthood and affect individuals throughout their lives. In fact, recent research suggests that up to 60% of children with ADHD will continue to experience symptoms in adulthood. However, the symptoms of ADHD may change as an individual matures. Children with ADHD may exhibit hyperactive and impulsive behaviors, while adults with ADHD may struggle more with inattention, organization, and time management. Adult ADHD can have a significant impact on various aspects of life, including work, relationships, and daily functioning.

Misconception 3: ADHD is caused by bad parenting or lack of discipline.

Another harmful misconception about ADHD is that it is caused by bad parenting or lack of discipline. This misconception can result in blame and shame being placed on parents or individuals with ADHD themselves, which is not only inaccurate but also unfair. ADHD is a complex condition with multiple contributing factors, including genetics, brain chemistry, and environmental influences. While parenting strategies and environmental factors can impact ADHD symptoms, they do not cause ADHD. In fact, research has shown that ADHD is highly heritable, with a strong genetic component. It is essential to understand that ADHD is not a result of poor parenting or lack of discipline, but rather a neurodevelopmental disorder that requires appropriate diagnosis and treatment.

Misconception 4: People with ADHD are just lazy or unmotivated.

It is a common misconception that people with ADHD are lazy or unmotivated, and that their difficulties with attention and focus are simply a result of a lack of effort or willpower. However, this is not the case. Individuals with ADHD often struggle with executive functions, which are cognitive processes that are responsible for planning, organizing, initiating tasks, and self-regulating behavior. These challenges can result in difficulties with time management, task initiation, and completion, which may be mistaken for laziness or lack of motivation. In reality, individuals with ADHD often put in significant effort to manage their symptoms and succeed in various aspects of life.

Misconception 5: Medication is the only treatment for ADHD.

While medication can be an effective treatment option for ADHD, it is not the only treatment available. Behavioral therapy, psychoeducation, and environmental modifications are also important components of a comprehensive treatment plan for ADHD. Behavioral therapy, such as cognitive-behavioral therapy (CBT), can help individuals with ADHD develop strategies to manage their symptoms, improve organizational skills, and learn coping mechanisms. Psychoeducation, which involves educating individuals with ADHD and their families about the condition, can help

Recognizing the symptoms of ADHD

Attention-Deficit/Hyperactivity Disorder (ADHD) is a neurodevelopmental disorder that commonly presents in childhood, but can also persist into adulthood. The symptoms of ADHD can vary depending on the individual and can be categorized into three main types: inattention, hyperactivity, and impulsivity. Here are some common symptoms of ADHD:

Inattention symptoms:
Difficulty paying attention to details or making careless mistakes in schoolwork or tasks.
Trouble staying focused during tasks or activities, including difficulty organizing and completing tasks.
Forgetfulness in daily activities, such as losing personal items like keys or forgetting appointments or deadlines.
Difficulty following instructions or listening when spoken to directly.

Struggling with organization and time management skills.

Hyperactivity symptoms:

Feeling restless or constantly "on the go" and having difficulty sitting still, particularly in situations where it is expected.

Fidgeting or squirming in seat.

Talking excessively or interrupting others during conversations or activities.

Difficulty engaging in quiet leisure activities.

Impulsivity symptoms:

Acting on impulse without considering consequences, such as blurting out answers in class or interrupting others.

Difficulty waiting for their turn in a conversation or in a queue.

Impatience and difficulty delaying gratification.

It's important to note that not everyone with ADHD will exhibit all of these symptoms, and the severity and presentation of symptoms can vary widely. Additionally, these symptoms should be pervasive, persistent, and significantly impact daily functioning in multiple settings, such as at home, school, work, or social settings, in order to meet the criteria for an ADHD diagnosis. If you suspect that you or someone you know may have ADHD, it's important to seek a professional evaluation from a qualified healthcare provider, such as a psychiatrist or psychologist, for an accurate diagnosis and appropriate management.

Understanding the impact of ADHD on self-esteem

ADHD (Attention-Deficit/Hyperactivity Disorder) is a neurodevelopmental disorder that can significantly impact an individual's self-esteem. Self-esteem refers to a person's perception of their self-worth, and it plays a crucial role in shaping their thoughts, feelings, and behaviors. ADHD can affect self-esteem in several ways:

Academic and Professional Challenges: Individuals with ADHD often face challenges with attention, focus, organization, and impulsivity, which can negatively impact their academic or professional performance. Struggling with school or work can lead to feelings of inadequacy, failure, and low self-esteem.

Social Difficulties: ADHD symptoms such as impulsivity, hyperactivity, and inattention can also affect social interactions. Individuals with ADHD may struggle with forming and maintaining relationships, experiencing rejection or social isolation. These social challenges can lead to feelings of low self-worth, self-doubt, and reduced self-esteem.

Internalizing Negative Feedback: Individuals with ADHD may receive negative feedback from teachers, peers, or employers due to their symptoms affecting their performance. This can lead to internalizing these negative messages and developing a negative perception of oneself, contributing to lower self-esteem.

Chronic Struggles with Self-Regulation: Managing time, staying organized, and controlling impulses can be challenging for individuals with ADHD. This chronic struggle with self-regulation can result in feelings of frustration, disappointment, and self-blame, leading to a negative impact on self-esteem.

Internal Shame and Stigma: Due to the societal misconceptions and stigma surrounding ADHD, individuals with ADHD may internalize shame and negative self-perception. They may feel "different" or "broken," leading to lowered self-esteem and self-worth.

Self-Identity Challenges: ADHD can affect an individual's sense of self-identity. They may struggle with understanding and accepting their ADHD diagnosis, and may feel like they don't fit in with societal norms or expectations. This can lead to a sense of identity crisis and reduced self-esteem.

It's important to note that self-esteem can be influenced by many factors, and not everyone with ADHD will experience low self-esteem. However, the challenges posed by ADHD can impact an individual's perception of themselves, leading to negative effects on self-esteem. Seeking support from mental health professionals, developing coping strategies, and building a strong support system can be helpful in managing the impact of ADHD on self-esteem.

Chapter 2: Navigating Diagnosis and Treatment

The importance of getting a proper diagnosis

Getting a proper diagnosis of Attention-Deficit/Hyperactivity Disorder (ADHD) is crucial for several reasons. Here are some key points highlighting the importance of obtaining an accurate diagnosis for ADHD:

Accurate understanding of symptoms: ADHD is a neurodevelopmental disorder that affects attention, impulse control, and hyperactivity. However, its symptoms can also overlap with other conditions, such as anxiety, depression, or learning disabilities. An accurate diagnosis helps in differentiating ADHD from other conditions and provides a clear understanding of the specific symptoms experienced by the individual.

Tailored treatment plan: An accurate diagnosis allows for the development of a customized treatment plan. Treatment approaches for ADHD may include medication, therapy, behavior modification, and other interventions. However, the most effective treatment plan may vary depending on the individual's specific symptoms, age, and other factors. A proper diagnosis helps in identifying the most appropriate treatment strategies to manage the symptoms effectively.

Access to appropriate support: With an accurate diagnosis, individuals with ADHD can access appropriate support systems. This may include working with healthcare professionals, educators, and other specialists who can provide guidance and support in managing ADHD symptoms. It can also facilitate accommodations and support in educational and workplace settings to optimize functioning and success.

Understanding of challenges and strengths: An accurate diagnosis helps individuals with ADHD gain a better understanding of their challenges and strengths. It provides validation for their struggles and helps them make sense of their experiences. This knowledge can empower individuals with ADHD to develop coping strategies, build self-awareness, and leverage their strengths for personal growth and success.

Avoidance of unnecessary interventions: Misdiagnosis or lack of diagnosis may result in inappropriate or unnecessary interventions. For example, without a proper ADHD diagnosis, individuals may be treated for other conditions that do not address the underlying ADHD symptoms. This can lead to ineffective treatment, frustration, and delayed progress in managing ADHD-related challenges.

Long-term outcomes: Untreated ADHD can have significant consequences on various aspects of an individual's life, including academics, work, relationships, and overall quality of life. However, with proper diagnosis and timely intervention, individuals with ADHD can learn effective strategies to manage their symptoms, improve their functioning, and achieve better long-term outcomes.

In conclusion, obtaining a proper diagnosis of ADHD is critical for accurate understanding of symptoms, tailored treatment planning, access to appropriate support, understanding of challenges and strengths, avoidance of unnecessary interventions, and improved long-term outcomes. If you suspect you or someone you know may have ADHD, it is essential to seek professional evaluation from a qualified healthcare provider for an accurate diagnosis and appropriate management.

Understanding different treatment options for ADHD

There are several different treatment options available for managing ADHD, which can be broadly categorized into three main approaches: behavioral therapy, medication, and lifestyle changes. Let's explore each of these options in more detail:

Behavioral Therapy: Behavioral therapy, also known as psychosocial interventions, focuses on modifying behaviors and improving skills related to managing ADHD symptoms. This can include various techniques such as cognitive-behavioral therapy (CBT), social skills training, parent training, and school-based interventions. Behavioral therapy aims to improve self-control, impulse management, organizational skills, time management, and problem-solving abilities. It can be particularly effective for children and adolescents with ADHD, but can also be beneficial for adults.

Medication: Medication is a common treatment approach for managing ADHD symptoms. Stimulant medications, such as methylphenidate (e.g., Ritalin, Concerta) and amphetamine (e.g., Adderall, Vyvanse), are commonly prescribed for ADHD. These medications help to improve attention, focus, impulse control, and reduce hyperactivity. Non-stimulant medications, such as atomoxetine (Strattera) and guanfacine (Intuniv), may also be prescribed, especially for individuals who cannot tolerate stimulants or have a history of substance abuse. Medication should always be prescribed and monitored by a qualified healthcare professional.

Lifestyle Changes: Making certain lifestyle changes can also help manage ADHD symptoms. This can include creating a structured environment with consistent routines, setting up a clear schedule, minimizing distractions, and organizing tasks and belongings. Regular exercise, healthy sleep habits, and a balanced diet can also support overall well-being and potentially help with ADHD symptoms. Some individuals with ADHD may also benefit from assistive technologies, such as reminder apps, timers, or noise-cancelling headphones.

It's important to note that the most effective treatment plan for ADHD often involves a combination of these approaches, tailored to the individual's unique needs and circumstances. Treatment plans should be developed in consultation with qualified healthcare professionals, such as psychiatrists, psychologists, or other healthcare providers with expertise in

ADHD. They can assess symptoms, provide accurate diagnoses, and recommend appropriate treatments based on the individual's age, severity of symptoms, medical history, and personal preferences.

Managing medication and its effects

Managing medication for ADHD (Attention Deficit Hyperactivity Disorder) involves several important aspects, including proper usage of medication, monitoring for side effects, and evaluating its effectiveness. Here are some key points to consider when managing medication for ADHD:

Follow the prescribed dosage and timing: It is crucial to take the medication exactly as prescribed by your healthcare provider. Follow the recommended dosage and timing instructions to ensure the medication is effective and safe.

Be aware of potential side effects: ADHD medications, such as stimulants (e.g., methylphenidate, amphetamine) and non-stimulants (e.g., atomoxetine, guanfacine), can have side effects. Common side effects may include decreased appetite, difficulty sleeping, increased heart rate, and increased blood pressure. Be aware of these potential side effects and communicate any concerns or issues to your healthcare provider promptly.

Monitor for changes in symptoms: Pay close attention to any changes in ADHD symptoms, both positive and negative, after starting medication. Keep a journal to track any improvements or changes in behavior, mood, focus, and attention. If you notice any significant changes or concerns, consult your healthcare provider for further evaluation and potential adjustments to the medication regimen.

Communicate with your healthcare provider: It is essential to maintain regular communication with your healthcare provider when managing ADHD medication. Inform them about any changes in symptoms, side effects, or concerns. Your healthcare provider may need to adjust the dosage or change the medication based on your response to treatment.

Consider behavioral interventions: Medication is just one component of a comprehensive treatment plan for ADHD. Behavioral interventions, such as therapy, counseling, and strategies to improve organization and time management skills, can also be effective in managing ADHD symptoms. Combining medication with behavioral interventions may yield better outcomes.

Educate yourself and your loved ones: It's important to understand ADHD and its treatment options thoroughly. Educate yourself and your loved ones about the medication being used, including its benefits, risks, and potential side effects. This will help you make informed decisions and manage ADHD effectively.

Follow lifestyle recommendations: In addition to medication, following healthy lifestyle recommendations can also support the management of ADHD. These may include regular exercise, adequate sleep, a healthy diet, and stress management techniques. Discuss with your healthcare provider for personalized lifestyle recommendations.

Remember that managing ADHD medication is an ongoing process that requires close collaboration with your healthcare provider. Regular follow-ups, open communication, and careful monitoring of symptoms and side effects are key to effectively managing medication for ADHD.

Developing a support system for coping with ADHD

Developing a support system for coping with ADHD (Attention Deficit Hyperactivity Disorder) can be beneficial in managing the challenges associated with the condition. Here are some steps you can take to create a support system for coping with ADHD:

Educate Yourself: Learn as much as you can about ADHD. Understand the symptoms, causes, and treatments. Educate yourself about different strategies and coping mechanisms that can help manage ADHD symptoms.

Seek Professional Help: Consult with a qualified healthcare professional, such as a psychiatrist or psychologist, who can diagnose ADHD and provide guidance on treatment options. They may recommend medication, therapy, or a combination of both.

Build a Team: Surround yourself with supportive individuals who can provide encouragement and understanding. This may include family members, friends, teachers, mentors, or support groups. These individuals can offer emotional support, practical advice, and help you stay accountable to your goals.

Develop Coping Strategies: Work with your healthcare professional to develop coping strategies that are tailored to your specific needs. This may include techniques to improve time management, organization, and impulse control. It may also involve developing strategies to manage emotional regulation and improve focus.

Create a Structured Routine: Establishing a routine can help with managing ADHD symptoms. Create a schedule that includes regular sleep patterns, consistent meal times, and dedicated times for work, study, and relaxation. Stick to the routine as much as possible to create stability and structure in your daily life.

Practice Self-Care: Taking care of your physical and mental health is crucial in managing ADHD. Make sure to get regular exercise, eat a healthy diet, and get enough sleep. Practice stress-management techniques such as mindfulness, meditation, and deep breathing exercises to help manage stress and anxiety.

Utilize Assistive Tools: There are various tools and technologies available that can help individuals with ADHD manage their symptoms. These may include digital calendars, task management apps, reminders, timers, and noise-cancelling headphones. Experiment with different tools and find what works best for you.

Advocate for Yourself: Be proactive in advocating for your needs. Communicate with your healthcare professional, teachers, employers, and loved ones about your challenges and what support you require. Seek accommodations if necessary, such as extended deadlines or modified work environments, to help you succeed.

Remember that managing ADHD is a lifelong journey, and it's important to be patient with yourself. Surrounding yourself with a supportive system can greatly improve your ability to cope with ADHD and lead a fulfilling life.

Chapter 3: Embracing Self-Care

Understanding the concept of self-care

Self-care is the practice of taking intentional actions to prioritize and maintain one's physical, mental, and emotional well-being. It involves engaging in activities that promote self-nurturing, self-soothing, and self-preservation, with the goal of enhancing overall health and resilience.

Self-care is essential for maintaining balance and managing stress in daily life. It involves recognizing and addressing one's own needs, setting healthy boundaries, and making time for self-reflection and self-improvement. Self-care is not selfish; it is a vital component of self-preservation and maintaining optimal functioning in various aspects of life, including work, relationships, and personal growth.

Self-care can take many different forms, and it can vary depending on individual preferences and circumstances. It may include physical self-care, such as getting regular exercise, eating a balanced diet, getting enough sleep, and attending to one's personal hygiene. It may also involve mental and emotional self-care, such as engaging in relaxation techniques, practicing mindfulness or meditation, seeking support from trusted friends or professionals, and engaging in activities that bring joy and fulfillment.

Setting healthy boundaries is also an important aspect of self-care. This means learning to say "no" when necessary, delegating tasks when possible, and not overextending oneself beyond what is reasonable or healthy. Boundaries help protect one's physical, mental, and emotional well-being and prevent burnout.

Practicing self-compassion is also a key element of self-care. It involves treating oneself with kindness, understanding, and patience, and reframing negative self-talk into more positive and constructive thoughts. Self-compassion involves acknowledging one's imperfections and mistakes without harsh self-judgment, and practicing self-forgiveness and self-acceptance.

Overall, self-care is about making intentional choices to prioritize and care for oneself, recognizing that self-care is not only important, but also necessary for overall well-being. By taking care of oneself, individuals can better manage stress, enhance their resilience, and live a more balanced and fulfilling life.

Recognizing the importance of self-care for teens with ADHD

Managing ADHD can be challenging, and self-care plays a crucial role in promoting overall well-being and mitigating the impact of ADHD symptoms on a teenager's daily life. Here are some key reasons why self-care is vital for teens with ADHD:

Managing symptoms: Self-care strategies such as regular exercise, healthy eating, sufficient sleep, and stress reduction techniques can help teens with ADHD manage their symptoms better. Physical activity can help reduce hyperactivity and impulsivity, while proper nutrition and sleep can support cognitive function and emotional regulation. Stress reduction techniques, such as mindfulness or relaxation exercises, can also help teens with ADHD cope with the challenges of daily life and reduce the impact of stress on their symptoms.

Enhancing focus and productivity: ADHD often impacts a teenager's ability to focus and complete tasks efficiently. Engaging in self-care activities that promote relaxation and stress reduction, such as meditation or spending time in nature, can help improve focus and concentration. Additionally, maintaining a healthy lifestyle, including regular exercise and a balanced diet, can support cognitive function and increase productivity.

Boosting self-esteem and self-confidence: Teens with ADHD may struggle with self-esteem and self-confidence due to challenges associated with their condition, such as academic difficulties or social interactions. Engaging in self-care activities that promote self-acceptance, self-compassion, and self-confidence, such as engaging in hobbies or activities they enjoy, practicing self-affirmation, or seeking support from trusted individuals, can help boost their self-esteem and self-confidence.

Preventing burnout: Managing the symptoms of ADHD can be demanding and overwhelming, and teens with ADHD may be at risk of experiencing burnout. Practicing self-care and setting healthy boundaries can help prevent burnout by ensuring that teens with ADHD take the time to rest, relax, and recharge. This can include setting limits on activities, prioritizing self-care activities, and learning to say no when needed.

Promoting emotional well-being: ADHD can impact emotional regulation and contribute to mood swings, impulsivity, and irritability. Engaging in self-care activities that promote emotional well-being, such as engaging in hobbies, spending time with supportive friends and family, seeking therapy or counseling, or practicing mindfulness, can help teens with ADHD manage their emotions and reduce the impact of emotional dysregulation on their daily lives.

In conclusion, self-care is crucial for teens with ADHD to manage their symptoms, enhance focus and productivity, boost self-esteem and self-confidence, prevent burnout, and promote emotional well-being. Encouraging and supporting teens with ADHD in developing self-care habits can be beneficial for their overall well-being and their ability to effectively manage their condition. It's important to work with healthcare professionals, such as doctors or therapists, to develop a comprehensive self-care plan that meets the unique needs of each individual with ADHD.

Developing healthy habits and routines

Developing healthy habits and routines is crucial for maintaining overall well-being and leading a fulfilling life. Here are some tips to help you establish healthy habits and routines:

Set specific goals: Start by setting clear, measurable, and realistic goals that are aligned with your values and priorities. Whether it's exercising regularly, eating a balanced diet, getting enough sleep, or practicing mindfulness, having specific goals in mind will help you stay focused and motivated.

Create a plan: Once you have identified your goals, create a plan of action to achieve them. Break down your goals into smaller, manageable steps and set a timeline for each step. Having a plan in place will help you stay organized and track your progress.

Be consistent: Consistency is key when it comes to developing healthy habits and routines. Try to establish a consistent schedule and stick to it as much as possible. Consistency helps your body and mind to adapt to new habits and makes them easier to maintain over time.

Start small: Instead of trying to overhaul your entire lifestyle all at once, start with small, achievable changes. For example, if you want to exercise more, begin with short workouts or brisk walks, and gradually increase the intensity and duration. Starting small allows you to build momentum and increases the likelihood of success.

Find motivation: Find what motivates you and use it to your advantage. It could be the benefits of a healthy lifestyle, the sense of accomplishment, or the support of loved ones. When you feel motivated, it's easier to stay committed to your healthy habits and routines.

Be flexible: It's important to be flexible and adaptable as you develop healthy habits and routines. Life can be unpredictable, and there may be times when you face setbacks or obstacles. When that happens, instead of getting discouraged, find ways to adjust your plans and keep moving forward.

Prioritize self-care: Taking care of yourself is essential for developing healthy habits and routines. Make sure to prioritize self-care by taking time for relaxation, self-reflection, and practicing good mental health habits, such as managing stress and seeking support when needed.

Surround yourself with support: Surround yourself with people who support your efforts to develop healthy habits and routines. Having a support system can provide accountability, encouragement, and motivation to stick to your goals.

Track your progress: Keep track of your progress to stay motivated and see how far you've come. You can use a journal, an app, or any other method that works for you. Celebrate your achievements, and use any setbacks as opportunities to learn and improve.

Remember that developing healthy habits and routines takes time and effort. Be patient with yourself and give yourself grace during the process. With consistent effort and determination, you can establish healthy habits and routines that will positively impact your physical, mental, and emotional well-being.

Coping strategies for managing stress and overwhelm

Coping strategies for managing stress and overwhelm can vary depending on individual preferences and circumstances.

Here are some general coping strategies that may be helpful:

Practice mindfulness: Mindfulness involves paying attention to the present moment without judgment. You can practice mindfulness through meditation, deep breathing exercises, or simply by focusing your attention on your surroundings, sensations, and thoughts. Mindfulness can help you become more aware of your stressors and manage them with a calm and centered mindset.

Engage in physical activity: Physical activity, such as exercise or sports, can help reduce stress and anxiety by releasing endorphins, which are natural mood-enhancing chemicals in the brain. Regular physical activity can also improve your overall well-being and help you better cope with stress.

Prioritize self-care: Taking care of yourself is crucial when managing stress and overwhelm. Make sure to prioritize self-care activities such as getting enough sleep, eating healthy meals, staying hydrated, and engaging in activities that you enjoy and that help you relax.

Practice time management: Feeling overwhelmed can often be a result of poor time management. Create a schedule or to-do list to prioritize tasks and break them down into smaller, more manageable steps. This can help you stay organized, focused, and reduce feelings of overwhelm.

Seek support from others: Don't be afraid to reach out to trusted friends, family members, or a therapist for support. Talking to someone about your stressors and concerns can provide perspective, validation, and emotional support.

Set healthy boundaries: It's important to set healthy boundaries to protect your time, energy, and mental well-being. Learn to say "no" when you need to and establish clear boundaries with work, social commitments, and other responsibilities to avoid becoming overwhelmed.

Practice relaxation techniques: Relaxation techniques, such as deep breathing, progressive muscle relaxation, or guided imagery, can help you reduce stress and promote relaxation. Incorporate these techniques into your daily routine to manage stress and overwhelm effectively.

Limit exposure to stressors: Identify sources of stress in your life and take steps to limit your exposure to them. This may involve reducing time spent on social media, setting limits on news consumption, or avoiding stressful situations whenever possible.

Practice good communication: Clear and effective communication can help you express your needs, set expectations, and reduce misunderstandings that can contribute to stress. Improve your communication skills by actively listening, expressing yourself assertively, and resolving conflicts in a healthy manner.

Practice positive self-talk: Monitor your self-talk and challenge negative or self-deprecating thoughts. Replace them with positive and affirming thoughts. Cultivating a positive mindset can help you better cope with stress and overwhelm.

Remember that coping strategies are individual, and it's important to find what works best for you. If you find that stress and overwhelm persist despite your efforts, consider seeking professional help from a therapist or counselor.

Chapter 4: Enhancing Executive Functioning Skills

Understanding the role of executive functioning in ADHD

Executive functioning refers to a set of cognitive processes that are responsible for managing and coordinating various cognitive and behavioral tasks in order to achieve goals effectively. These processes are commonly associated with the prefrontal cortex of the brain and are crucial for self-regulation, decision-making, problem-solving, attention, impulse control, planning, organization, working memory, and emotional regulation.

In individuals with ADHD (Attention Deficit Hyperactivity Disorder), executive functioning deficits are a hallmark feature. ADHD is a neurodevelopmental disorder that affects both children and adults, characterized by persistent difficulties with attention, hyperactivity, and impulsivity. Executive functioning deficits are believed to underlie many of the challenges experienced by individuals with ADHD.

Some key roles of executive functioning in ADHD include:

Attention: Executive functioning deficits in ADHD can lead to difficulties in sustaining attention, shifting attention, and selectively focusing on relevant information. Individuals with ADHD may struggle with distractions, have trouble following instructions, and have difficulty staying engaged in tasks that require sustained attention, such as studying or listening to lectures.

Impulse control: Poor impulse control is a common symptom of ADHD, which can result in impulsive behaviors such as interrupting others, blurting out answers, or acting without thinking. Executive functioning deficits in ADHD can lead to difficulties in inhibiting impulsive responses and considering consequences before acting.

Working memory: Working memory refers to the ability to hold and manipulate information in mind over short periods of time. Executive functioning deficits in ADHD can result in poor working memory, making it challenging for individuals to remember and use information in the moment, such as following multi-step instructions or solving complex problems.

Planning and organization: Executive functioning deficits in ADHD can affect an individual's ability to plan and organize tasks, set goals, initiate tasks, and complete them in a timely manner. Individuals with ADHD may struggle with prioritizing tasks, managing time, and organizing their environment, leading to difficulties with task completion and meeting deadlines.

Emotional regulation: Executive functioning deficits in ADHD can also impact an individual's ability to regulate emotions effectively. Individuals with ADHD may have difficulty managing frustration, anger, or impatience, and may exhibit emotional outbursts or mood swings.

It's important to note that executive functioning deficits in ADHD can vary widely from person to person and can change over time. However, understanding the role of executive functioning in ADHD can help individuals with ADHD, their families, and educators develop strategies and interventions to support the management of ADHD symptoms and improve daily functioning. Interventions may include behavioral strategies, psychoeducation, medication, and other supportive measures tailored to the individual's unique needs. Consulting with a qualified healthcare professional or a licensed mental health provider is recommended for accurate assessment and appropriate management of ADHD symptoms.

Developing strategies for improving time management

Time management is a crucial skill for being productive and achieving your goals. Here are some strategies to improve time management:

Set clear goals: Start by defining your short-term and long-term goals. These goals will serve as a roadmap for your tasks and activities, helping you prioritize and allocate time accordingly.

Prioritize tasks: Make a to-do list and prioritize tasks based on their importance and urgency. Focus on completing the most important and time-sensitive tasks first.

Plan ahead: Create a daily or weekly schedule to plan your tasks in advance. Set aside dedicated time slots for specific activities and stick to your schedule as much as possible.

Avoid multitasking: Multitasking can be counterproductive as it can reduce overall efficiency. Instead, focus on one task at a time and complete it before moving on to the next one.

Delegate tasks: If possible, delegate tasks to others to free up your time for more important or higher-value activities. Learn to trust and rely on your team or colleagues to share the workload.

Minimize distractions: Identify and eliminate or minimize distractions that hinder your productivity, such as social media, unnecessary notifications, or interruptions. Consider using productivity tools or apps to block distractions during work hours.

Practice time blocking: Time blocking involves scheduling specific time blocks for different tasks or activities. This can help you stay focused and disciplined, as well as ensure that you allocate enough time for each task.

Learn to say no: It's important to learn to say no to non-essential tasks or activities that do not align with your priorities or goals. This will help you avoid overcommitting and manage your time more effectively.

Take breaks: Taking regular breaks can actually improve productivity. Schedule short breaks during your work hours to rest and recharge, so you can maintain focus and energy throughout the day.

Review and adjust: Regularly review your progress and adjust your time management strategies as needed. Reflect on what works and what doesn't, and make necessary changes to optimize your time management approach.

Remember that time management is a skill that takes practice and consistency. By implementing these strategies and making them a part of your routine, you can improve your time management skills and become more productive in achieving your goals.

Enhancing organizational skills and study habits

Enhancing organizational skills and study habits is crucial for academic success and overall productivity. Here are some tips to improve organizational skills and study habits:

Create a study schedule: Plan a schedule that includes dedicated time for studying, reviewing, and completing assignments. Set specific goals for each study session, and stick to the schedule as much as possible.

Use a planner or digital tools: Keep track of important deadlines, assignments, and exams using a planner or digital tools such as calendars, task management apps, or online study platforms. Use these tools to prioritize tasks and stay organized.

Declutter your study space: A clean and organized study environment can help improve focus and productivity. Keep your study area tidy and free from distractions, and only have essential study materials within reach.

Break tasks into smaller chunks: Large tasks or assignments can be overwhelming. Break them down into smaller, more manageable tasks, and work on them systematically. This can help you avoid procrastination and make progress steadily.

Prioritize tasks: Determine which tasks are most important and prioritize them accordingly. Focus on completing high-priority tasks first to ensure you are making progress on the most critical assignments or studying for the most significant exams.

Take regular breaks: Taking short breaks during study sessions can actually boost productivity. Use the Pomodoro Technique, where you work for a focused period of time (e.g., 25 minutes) and then take a short break (e.g., 5 minutes). Repeat this cycle to maintain focus and motivation.

Use effective study techniques: Experiment with different study techniques to find what works best for you. Some popular techniques include active reading, summarizing information in your own words, creating flashcards, and teaching the material to someone else.

Review regularly: Regularly review your notes, assignments, and study materials to reinforce learning and help with retention. Set aside time for review sessions in your study schedule.

Seek help when needed: Don't hesitate to seek help from teachers, tutors, or peers if you are struggling with understanding the material or organizing your tasks. They can provide valuable guidance and support.

Stay motivated and disciplined: Improving organizational skills and study habits requires discipline and consistency. Stay motivated by setting goals, rewarding yourself for achievements, and maintaining a positive mindset.

Remember, enhancing organizational skills and study habits takes time and effort, so be patient with yourself. With consistent practice and determination, you can develop effective organizational skills and study habits that will benefit you throughout your academic and professional life.

Managing impulsivity and improving decision-making skills

Managing impulsivity and improving decision-making skills are important life skills that can lead to better outcomes and improved overall well-being. Here are some tips to help you in this regard:

Pause and reflect: When faced with a decision or an impulse to act, take a moment to pause and reflect. Avoid acting on impulse without considering the potential consequences. Take deep breaths, count to ten, or give yourself a designated time frame to think before taking action.

Identify triggers: Understand what triggers impulsive behavior or poor decision-making in your life. Is it stress, emotions, peer pressure, or other external factors? Identifying triggers can help you be more mindful and prepared when faced with situations that may lead to impulsive actions.

Practice self-awareness: Develop self-awareness by being in tune with your thoughts, feelings, and emotions. Pay attention to your internal state and how it may impact your decision-making. Being self-aware can help you recognize impulsive tendencies and take steps to manage them.

Evaluate pros and cons: When making decisions, weigh the pros and cons of each option. Consider the potential outcomes, risks, and benefits. This can help you make more informed decisions rather than succumbing to impulsive choices.

Seek input from others: Seek input from trusted friends, family, or mentors before making important decisions. Getting a fresh perspective can provide valuable insights and help you see things from different angles, which can aid in making better decisions.

Set goals and priorities: Establish clear goals and priorities in your life. Having a sense of purpose and direction can guide your decision-making and reduce impulsive actions that may not align with your long-term objectives.

Practice delayed gratification: Learn to delay gratification by resisting impulsive urges for immediate rewards. Practice patience and discipline, and focus on long-term gains rather than short-term impulses.

Learn from mistakes: Acknowledge that mistakes are a part of life and an opportunity to learn and grow. When you make poor decisions or act impulsively, reflect on what went wrong and how you can improve in the future.

Develop a decision-making process: Create a structured decision-making process that involves gathering information, evaluating options, considering consequences, and making informed choices. Having a systematic approach can help you make more rational decisions and reduce impulsive behavior.

Practice mindfulness: Mindfulness techniques, such as meditation or mindfulness exercises, can help you develop better self-regulation and improve decision-making skills. Being present in the moment and non-judgmentally observing your thoughts and emotions can increase self-awareness and enable more thoughtful decision-making.

Remember, improving impulsivity and decision-making skills is a gradual process that requires practice and self-reflection. Be patient with yourself and celebrate small victories along the way. With time and effort, you can develop better decision-making habits and manage impulsivity effectively.

Chapter 5: Building Positive Relationships

Navigating social challenges associated with ADHD

As someone with ADHD, navigating social challenges can be difficult, but with some strategies and techniques, you can effectively manage them. Here are some tips:

Educate Yourself: Learn about ADHD and how it affects your social interactions. Understand the symptoms and challenges associated with ADHD, such as impulsivity, hyperactivity, and inattention. This knowledge will help you better understand your own behavior and responses in social situations.

Seek Support: Reach out to a trusted friend, family member, or therapist for support. Talking to someone about your challenges can provide you with emotional support and help you develop coping strategies.

Practice Self-Awareness: Be mindful of your own behavior in social situations. Pay attention to how ADHD affects your interactions with others, such as interrupting or getting distracted. Being self-aware can help you identify areas that need improvement and make adjustments accordingly.

Develop Social Skills: Practice and develop social skills, such as active listening, empathy, and non-verbal communication. These skills can help you build stronger relationships and improve your social interactions.

Use Time Management Strategies: ADHD can affect your ability to manage time effectively, leading to challenges with punctuality and meeting social commitments. Use strategies such as setting reminders, creating schedules, and using timers to help you stay organized and on track.

Communicate Openly: Be open and honest with others about your ADHD. Explain how it affects your social interactions and ask for their understanding and support. This can help you create a supportive environment where others are aware of your challenges and can provide accommodations if needed.

Develop Coping Strategies: Develop coping strategies that work for you in social situations. For example, if you struggle with impulsivity, practice taking a moment to pause and think before responding in conversations. If you have difficulty with attention, try using active listening techniques, such as repeating back what someone said to ensure you understand.

Manage Anxiety and Rejection Sensitivity: ADHD can be associated with anxiety and rejection sensitivity, which can affect social interactions. Practice relaxation techniques, such as deep breathing or mindfulness, to help manage anxiety. If rejection sensitivity is a challenge, consider working with a therapist to develop coping strategies.

Build a Supportive Social Network: Surround yourself with understanding and supportive friends, family, and peers who accept you for who you are. Having a supportive social network can provide a sense of belonging and help you navigate social challenges associated with ADHD.

Remember, managing social challenges associated with ADHD takes time and effort. Be patient with yourself, celebrate your successes, and seek professional help if needed. With the right strategies and support, you can develop strong social skills and build meaningful relationships.

Communicating effectively with peers, family, and teachers

Effective communication is crucial in various aspects of life, including interactions with peers, family, and teachers. Here are some tips for communicating effectively in these different contexts:

Be an active listener: Listening attentively to what others are saying is a fundamental aspect of effective communication. Pay attention to both the verbal and non-verbal cues of the speaker, such as their tone of voice, facial expressions, and body language. Avoid interrupting or forming judgments while the other person is speaking, and make sure to respond appropriately to their message.

Use clear and concise language: When expressing your thoughts or ideas, use clear and concise language to convey your message effectively. Avoid using jargon, slang, or complicated language that may confuse others. Be mindful of your tone and try to express yourself in a respectful and considerate manner.

Ask clarifying questions: If you're unsure about something or need further information, don't hesitate to ask clarifying questions. This shows that you're actively engaged in the conversation and interested in understanding the other person's perspective. It also helps to avoid misunderstandings and misinterpretations.

Express yourself assertively: Assertive communication involves expressing your thoughts, feelings, and needs in a respectful and confident manner, while also considering the feelings and opinions of others. Avoid being passive, where you may fail to express your thoughts, or aggressive, where you may come across as confrontational or disrespectful.

Show empathy and understanding: Empathy and understanding are crucial in building healthy relationships and effective communication. Try to see things from the other person's perspective and acknowledge their emotions and experiences. This helps in fostering mutual respect and trust in your interactions.

Practice non-violent communication: Non-violent communication is a communication style that focuses on expressing oneself honestly and empathetically, while also actively listening to others. It involves using "I" statements to express your feelings and needs, and refraining from blame, criticism, or judgment. It encourages open and honest communication, leading to better understanding and resolution of conflicts.

Be mindful of your body language: Non-verbal cues, such as facial expressions, gestures, and posture, play a significant role in communication. Be aware of your body language and try to maintain eye contact, use appropriate gestures, and convey openness through your posture. This helps in conveying sincerity and building trust in your interactions.

Practice patience and respect: Effective communication requires patience and respect. Allow others to express themselves fully without interrupting or rushing to respond. Avoid belittling or disrespecting others' opinions or ideas, even if you disagree with them. Remember that everyone has the right to express themselves and be heard.

Seek feedback: Feedback is an essential part of effective communication. Encourage open and honest feedback from your peers, family, and teachers to understand how you can improve your communication skills. Be open to receiving constructive criticism and work on areas that need improvement.

Practice active and positive communication: Lastly, practice active and positive communication in all your interactions. Be proactive in initiating conversations, express gratitude and appreciation when appropriate, and strive to maintain a positive and constructive tone in your communication.

Effective communication is a skill that can be developed with practice and awareness. By incorporating these tips into your interactions with peers, family, and teachers, you can enhance your communication skills and build stronger and healthier relationships.

Developing empathy and understanding in relationships

Empathy and understanding are key components of healthy and fulfilling relationships. They allow individuals to connect on a deeper level, build trust, and foster meaningful connections with others. Developing empathy and understanding in relationships requires practice and effort, but it can be achieved with intentional steps. Here are some ways to cultivate empathy and understanding in your relationships:

Active Listening: Actively listen to the other person without interrupting or formulating your response in your mind. Give them your full attention and show genuine interest in their perspective. This helps you understand their thoughts, feelings, and experiences without judgment.

Put Yourself in Their Shoes: Try to understand the other person's point of view by putting yourself in their shoes. Consider their background, experiences, and emotions. This helps you gain perspective and empathize with their emotions and experiences.

Validate Their Feelings: Acknowledge and validate the other person's feelings, even if you don't agree with them. Avoid dismissing or minimizing their emotions. Show empathy by expressing understanding and compassion towards their emotions.

Ask Open-Ended Questions: Ask open-ended questions that encourage the other person to share more about their thoughts and feelings. This helps you gain a deeper understanding of their perspective and emotions.

Manage Your Own Emotions: It's important to manage your own emotions when trying to develop empathy and understanding. Avoid reacting impulsively or emotionally. Take a step back, practice self-regulation, and approach the situation with a calm and composed mindset.

Practice Perspective-Taking: Try to see things from the other person's perspective. Imagine yourself in their situation and consider how you would feel and react. This helps you develop a broader understanding of their emotions and experiences.

Show Empathy and Compassion: Express empathy and compassion towards the other person's emotions and experiences. Offer comfort, support, and understanding. This creates a safe space for open communication and fosters trust in the relationship.

Cultivate Emotional Intelligence: Developing emotional intelligence, which includes self-awareness, self-regulation, empathy, and social skills, can greatly enhance your ability to understand and empathize with others in relationships.

Practice Forgiveness: Forgiveness is an important aspect of understanding and empathy in relationships. Practice forgiveness towards yourself and others for mistakes or hurtful actions. This helps in healing and moving forward with empathy and understanding.

Be Open to Learning and Growth: Be open to learning and growing in your relationships. Acknowledge that everyone has different perspectives and experiences, and be willing to broaden your understanding and empathy towards others.

Remember that developing empathy and understanding is an ongoing process that requires practice and effort. It's a skill that can be developed and refined over time, and it can greatly enhance your relationships and overall well-being.

Building a support network for managing ADHD

Building a support network is essential for managing ADHD (Attention-Deficit/Hyperactivity Disorder) effectively. Here are some steps you can take to build a support network for managing ADHD:

Educate Yourself: Start by learning as much as you can about ADHD. Understand the symptoms, challenges, and treatment options available. Knowledge is power, and being well-informed about ADHD will help you advocate for yourself or your loved one effectively.

Seek Professional Help: Consult with a qualified healthcare professional, such as a psychiatrist or psychologist, who specializes in ADHD. They can provide an accurate diagnosis, prescribe medication if needed, and offer guidance on managing symptoms.

Join Support Groups: Connecting with others who have ADHD can be tremendously helpful. Look for local or online support groups where you can share experiences, exchange tips, and receive emotional support. There are many online communities, forums, and social media groups dedicated to ADHD where you can find like-minded individuals.

Involve Family and Friends: Educate your family and close friends about ADHD. Help them understand the challenges you face, and ask for their support. Having a strong support system of loved ones who understand and empathize with your struggles can make a significant difference in managing ADHD.

Collaborate with Educators and Employers: If you or your loved one with ADHD is in school or employed, collaborate with educators or employers to create accommodations that can help manage symptoms. This may include additional time for assignments or tests, modified work environments, or other reasonable adjustments to support success.

Seek Professional Coaching: Consider working with an ADHD coach, who can provide guidance, strategies, and tools for managing ADHD in daily life. ADHD coaches can help with time management, organization, and goal-setting skills, and provide ongoing support and accountability.

Take Care of Yourself: Managing ADHD can be challenging, so it's crucial to prioritize self-care. Make sure you get enough sleep, eat a healthy diet, exercise regularly, and engage in stress-reducing activities such as meditation, mindfulness, or hobbies that you enjoy.

Remember, building a support network for managing ADHD is a process that takes time and effort. It's important to surround yourself with people who are understanding, supportive, and knowledgeable about ADHD. With the right support system in place, you can effectively manage ADHD and lead a fulfilling life.

Chapter 6: Thriving in School

Understanding the academic challenges associated with ADHD

ADHD, or attention deficit hyperactivity disorder, is a neurodevelopmental disorder that affects both children and adults. It is characterized by symptoms such as inattention, hyperactivity, and impulsivity. These symptoms can pose significant challenges in an academic setting, affecting various aspects of a person's academic life. Here are some academic challenges associated with ADHD:

Inattention and poor focus: One of the hallmark symptoms of ADHD is difficulty with sustained attention and focus. This can make it challenging for individuals with ADHD to concentrate on lectures, readings, or assignments for long periods of time. They may struggle to stay on task, become easily distracted, or have difficulty organizing and prioritizing tasks, leading to difficulties in completing assignments or studying effectively.

Impulsivity and poor decision-making: Impulsivity is another core symptom of ADHD, which can lead to poor decision-making in an academic context. Individuals with ADHD may have difficulty thinking through the consequences of their actions before acting, leading to impulsive decisions such as procrastination, rushing through assignments, or not carefully checking their work, which can result in lower quality work or mistakes.

Time management difficulties: Many individuals with ADHD struggle with time management, which can impact their academic performance. They may have difficulty estimating how long tasks will take or struggle with prioritizing assignments or studying effectively. This can result in missed deadlines, incomplete assignments, or cramming at the last minute, which can negatively impact academic success.

Organization and planning challenges: Organization and planning skills are important for academic success, but individuals with ADHD may struggle with these skills. They may have difficulty keeping track of assignments, managing materials, or organizing their thoughts when writing papers or taking exams. This can lead to difficulties in meeting deadlines, submitting assignments on time, or effectively studying for exams.

Social and behavioral challenges: ADHD can also impact social interactions and behavior in an academic setting. Individuals with ADHD may struggle with impulse control, leading to disruptions in class, difficulties following classroom rules, or problems with peers. This can result in social and behavioral consequences such as negative feedback from teachers or strained relationships with classmates, which can affect academic performance.

Low motivation and engagement: ADHD can also impact motivation and engagement in academic tasks. Individuals with ADHD may struggle with maintaining interest in assignments or lectures that do not capture their attention, leading to low motivation to complete tasks or actively participate in class. This can result in reduced academic performance and difficulty meeting academic expectations.

It's important to note that not all individuals with ADHD will experience the same academic challenges, as symptoms can vary widely from person to person. However, these challenges highlight some common areas that individuals with ADHD may struggle with in an academic setting. Proper diagnosis, treatment, and support, such as medication, therapy, and accommodations, can help individuals with ADHD better manage these challenges and achieve academic success. Working closely with educators, school counselors, or other support professionals can also be beneficial in addressing academic challenges associated with ADHD.

Strategies for staying focused and engaged in class

Staying focused and engaged in class is essential for effective learning. Here are some strategies that can help you stay on track:

Create a conducive learning environment: Choose a quiet, well-lit place to attend your classes, free from distractions such as noisy surroundings or unnecessary gadgets.

Set clear goals: Before each class, set specific goals for what you want to achieve during that session. It could be taking notes, asking questions, or participating in discussions. Having clear objectives will help you stay focused and engaged.

Take breaks: Sitting for long periods can lead to decreased focus and attention. Take short breaks during longer classes to stretch, walk around, or do a quick mental reset to keep yourself engaged.

Actively participate: Participate in class discussions, ask questions, and share your thoughts. Active engagement not only keeps you focused but also reinforces your learning.

Take organized notes: Taking notes helps you process and retain information. Develop a note-taking system that works for you, whether it's handwritten or digital, and review your notes regularly to reinforce your understanding.

Minimize distractions: Turn off notifications on your phone or other electronic devices, close irrelevant tabs on your computer, and avoid multitasking. Minimizing distractions will help you stay focused on the class material.

Use different learning modalities: Engage in different ways of learning, such as visual, auditory, or kinesthetic, to keep yourself engaged. For example, if you're a visual learner, use diagrams or illustrations to reinforce your understanding.

Time management: Manage your time effectively by prioritizing your tasks and allocating specific time slots for class attendance, studying, and other activities. Avoid procrastination to prevent last-minute cramming or distractions during class time.

Get enough rest and eat well: Proper sleep and nutrition are essential for cognitive function. Make sure to get enough sleep and eat nutritious meals to keep your brain sharp and focused during class.

Stay motivated: Stay motivated by reminding yourself of the importance of the class material and how it aligns with your overall goals. Find ways to make the material relevant and interesting to you, which will help you stay engaged and focused.

Remember, staying focused and engaged in class requires discipline and effort, but it is crucial for effective learning. By implementing these strategies, you can improve your ability to stay focused and actively participate in class, leading to a better understanding of the material and better academic performance.

Managing homework and assignments effectively

Managing homework and assignments effectively is essential for academic success. Here are some tips to help you manage your homework and assignments efficiently:

Create a schedule: Start by creating a schedule that outlines all of your assignments and homework deadlines. Use a digital calendar or a planner to keep track of due dates, and prioritize tasks based on urgency and importance.

Break tasks into smaller, manageable chunks: Large assignments or projects can feel overwhelming, so break them down into smaller, more manageable tasks. This will help you avoid procrastination and make steady progress.

Prioritize tasks: Determine which tasks are most important and need to be completed first. Prioritize assignments based on their due dates, importance, and complexity. Focus on completing high-priority tasks before moving on to lower-priority ones.

Avoid multitasking: Trying to do multiple tasks at once can actually decrease productivity. Instead, focus on one task at a time and give it your full attention. This will help you complete tasks more efficiently and with better quality.

Create a productive study environment: Find a quiet and well-lit place to study that is free from distractions. Keep all necessary materials, such as textbooks, notebooks, and reference materials, within easy reach. Minimize distractions like social media, and use tools like website blockers if needed.

Set specific goals: Set specific goals for each homework or assignment session. For example, you might aim to complete a certain number of math problems or write a specific number of paragraphs for an essay. Having clear goals will help you stay focused and motivated.

Take regular breaks: Taking short breaks during your study or homework sessions can help improve focus and productivity. Avoid studying or working for long stretches without breaks, as it can lead to burnout and decreased effectiveness.

Seek help when needed: Don't hesitate to ask for help when you need it. If you're struggling with a particular assignment or concept, seek guidance from your teacher, classmates, or tutors. Asking for help can save you time and help you understand the material better.

Stay organized: Keep your assignments, notes, and study materials organized. Use folders or binders to store your papers and digital folders to store electronic documents. This will help you quickly locate what you need when you're working on assignments.

Avoid procrastination: Procrastination can lead to unnecessary stress and poor-quality work. Practice self-discipline and avoid putting off assignments until the last minute. Break tasks into smaller chunks and work on them consistently over time to avoid procrastination.

By following these tips, you can effectively manage your homework and assignments, stay organized, and achieve academic success. Remember to stay focused, prioritize tasks, seek help when needed, and practice good time management skills.

Advocating for accommodations and support in school

Advocating for accommodations and support in school can be a critical process for ensuring that students with special needs or disabilities have equal access to education. Here are some steps you can take to effectively advocate for accommodations and support in school:

Understand your rights: Familiarize yourself with the laws and regulations that protect the rights of students with disabilities, such as the Individuals with Disabilities Education Act (IDEA) and Section 504 of the Rehabilitation Act. These laws outline the rights of students with disabilities to receive appropriate accommodations and support in school.

Gather information: Collect relevant information about your child's disability, including any medical or educational evaluations, assessments, or reports that support the need for accommodations and support. This can provide you with evidence to support your advocacy efforts.

Communicate with school staff: Establish open lines of communication with your child's teachers, counselors, and school administrators. Share information about your child's disability and specific needs, and discuss potential accommodations and support that may be necessary. Be proactive in advocating for your child's needs and expressing your concerns.

Develop an Individualized Education Program (IEP) or Section 504 Plan: Work with the school's special education team to develop an IEP or Section 504 Plan for your child. These plans outline the specific accommodations, modifications, and support services that your child will receive in school. Review the plans regularly and ensure that they are being implemented effectively.

Attend meetings and be prepared: Attend all relevant meetings, such as IEP meetings or Section 504 Plan meetings, and come prepared. Bring copies of relevant documents, take notes during the meetings, and ask questions to clarify any information or decisions. Be an active participant in the process.

Seek support: If you encounter challenges or obstacles in advocating for accommodations and support, seek support from other sources. This can include working with advocacy organizations, seeking legal advice, or collaborating with other parents of students with disabilities to share information and strategies.

Document and follow up: Keep records of all communication and documentation related to your advocacy efforts. Follow up with school staff to ensure that accommodations and support are being provided as agreed upon. If necessary, follow up with school administrators or district officials to address any concerns or issues.

Remember, advocating for accommodations and support in school may require persistence and determination. It's important to be prepared, informed, and proactive in advocating for the needs of your child. By working collaboratively with school staff and using the resources available to you, you can help ensure that your child receives the appropriate accommodations and support for their educational success.

Chapter 7: Managing Emotions and Building Resilience

Understanding the emotional challenges of ADHD

ADHD, or Attention-Deficit/Hyperactivity Disorder, is a neurodevelopmental disorder that affects both children and adults. In addition to the hallmark symptoms of inattention, hyperactivity, and impulsivity, ADHD can also present with a range of emotional challenges that can impact an individual's well-being and quality of life. Some of the emotional challenges commonly associated with ADHD include:

Frustration and irritability: ADHD can make it difficult for individuals to focus and complete tasks, leading to feelings of frustration and irritability. They may struggle with organizing their thoughts or managing their time effectively, which can exacerbate these emotions.

Low self-esteem: Many individuals with ADHD face challenges with school, work, and relationships due to their symptoms, which can result in lower self-esteem. They may feel inadequate or struggle with a sense of failure, leading to feelings of self-doubt and low self-worth.

Anxiety and stress: ADHD can cause individuals to feel anxious and stressed, as they may struggle with meeting deadlines, keeping up with responsibilities, and managing their impulsivity. The constant pressure to perform at the same level as their peers can be overwhelming and lead to increased anxiety.

Mood swings: ADHD can impact an individual's ability to regulate their emotions, leading to mood swings. They may experience intense emotions such as anger, frustration, or sadness, which can be triggered by their challenges with attention, impulsivity, and hyperactivity.

Rejection and social difficulties: Individuals with ADHD may face challenges in social settings due to their symptoms. They may struggle with maintaining attention during conversations, impulsively interrupting others, or having difficulty with social cues. This can lead to feelings of rejection, social isolation, and difficulty forming and maintaining meaningful relationships.

Depression: The emotional challenges of ADHD can contribute to the development of depression in some individuals. Struggling with symptoms such as inattention, impulsivity, and hyperactivity on a daily basis can be exhausting and overwhelming, leading to feelings of sadness, hopelessness, and loss of interest in activities.

It's important to note that the emotional challenges associated with ADHD can vary from person to person, and not everyone with ADHD will experience all of these challenges. However, it's crucial to recognize that the emotional impact of ADHD is significant and can have a profound effect on an individual's mental health and well-being. Seeking appropriate support, such as therapy, counseling, medication, and lifestyle modifications, can be helpful in managing these emotional challenges and improving overall quality of life for individuals with ADHD.

Coping with frustration, anger, and disappointment

Coping with frustration, anger, and disappointment can be challenging, but it's important to learn healthy ways to manage these emotions in order to maintain your well-being and relationships. Here are some tips on how to cope with frustration, anger, and disappointment:

Take a pause: When you start feeling frustrated, angry, or disappointed, take a moment to pause and reflect. Try to step back from the situation and give yourself some space to process your emotions before reacting impulsively.

Acknowledge and validate your emotions: It's okay to feel frustrated, angry, or disappointed. Acknowledge and validate your emotions without judgment. Allow yourself to experience these emotions without trying to suppress or deny them.

Practice self-care: Engage in self-care activities that help you relax and calm down, such as deep breathing, meditation, exercise, or spending time in nature. Taking care of your physical and mental well-being can help you better manage your emotions.

Express your emotions in a healthy way: Find healthy outlets to express your emotions, such as talking to a trusted friend, journaling, or engaging in creative activities. Avoid lashing out or bottling up your emotions, as it can lead to further frustration and anger.

Challenge negative thoughts: Often, frustration, anger, and disappointment are fueled by negative thoughts and perceptions. Challenge and reframe these negative thoughts by looking at the situation from different perspectives and considering alternative explanations.

Set realistic expectations: Frustration, anger, and disappointment can arise when our expectations are not met. It's important to set realistic expectations for yourself and others, and to recognize that not everything will go as planned.

Practice assertive communication: Instead of reacting impulsively out of frustration or anger, practice assertive communication skills. Clearly express your thoughts and feelings in a respectful manner, and actively listen to others' perspectives.

Seek support: If you find it difficult to cope with frustration, anger, or disappointment on your own, don't hesitate to seek support from a trusted friend, family member, or mental health professional. They can provide you with guidance, perspective, and tools to cope effectively.

Remember, coping with frustration, anger, and disappointment is a process that takes time and practice. Be patient with yourself, and give yourself the space and grace to navigate these emotions in a healthy and constructive way.

Building emotional resilience and self-regulation skills

Emotional resilience and self-regulation skills are essential for navigating the ups and downs of life with grace and adaptability. They allow you to effectively manage stress, regulate your emotions, and bounce back from setbacks. Here are some tips for building emotional resilience and self-regulation skills:

Develop self-awareness: Self-awareness is the foundation of emotional resilience and self-regulation. Take time to understand your emotions, thoughts, and behaviors. Pay attention to your triggers, patterns, and reactions in different situations. This self-awareness will help you recognize when you're feeling overwhelmed or stressed, and allow you to respond intentionally rather than react impulsively.

Practice mindfulness: Mindfulness is the practice of being present in the moment without judgment. It can help you become more aware of your emotions and thoughts without getting caught up in them. Regular mindfulness practices such as meditation, deep breathing, or body scans can help you develop better emotional regulation by allowing you to observe your emotions and thoughts from a distance, and choose how you want to respond to them.

Build healthy coping strategies: Developing healthy coping strategies can help you manage stress and regulate your emotions effectively. Identify healthy coping mechanisms that work for you, such as exercise, talking to a supportive friend, engaging in a hobby, or practicing relaxation techniques. Avoid unhealthy coping mechanisms like substance abuse or excessive screen time, as they can exacerbate emotional challenges in the long run.

Cultivate social support: Social support is crucial for emotional resilience. Surround yourself with a supportive network of friends, family, or a therapist who can provide you with empathy, understanding, and guidance during difficult times. Having someone to talk to and share your emotions can help you process them and gain perspective, which can contribute to better emotional regulation.

Develop problem-solving skills: Building strong problem-solving skills can help you navigate challenges effectively and reduce stress. When faced with difficult situations, try to identify the problem, brainstorm potential solutions, evaluate them, and implement the best course of action. Problem-solving can help you feel more in control and reduce the emotional burden, contributing to better emotional resilience.

Practice self-care: Taking care of yourself physically, mentally, and emotionally is essential for emotional resilience. Get enough sleep, eat a healthy diet, engage in regular exercise, and practice good hygiene. Take time for self-care activities that bring you joy and help you relax, such as reading, spending time in nature, or practicing hobbies. Taking care of yourself holistically can boost your emotional well-being and strengthen your resilience.

Foster a positive mindset: Cultivating a positive mindset can help you develop emotional resilience. Practice gratitude by focusing on the things in your life that you appreciate. Challenge negative thoughts and reframe them in a more positive or realistic light. Foster a growth mindset by viewing challenges as opportunities for growth and learning. A positive mindset can help you build resilience and approach difficulties with a more adaptive attitude.

Remember, building emotional resilience and self-regulation skills is a journey that requires practice and patience. Be kind to yourself and give yourself time to develop these skills. With consistent effort and practice, you can enhance your emotional resilience and enjoy better emotional well-being. If you find yourself struggling, consider seeking support from a mental health professional.

Developing healthy coping mechanisms for managing emotions

Developing healthy coping mechanisms for managing emotions is an important aspect of emotional well-being and mental health. Here are some strategies that can help you develop healthy coping mechanisms for managing emotions:

Mindfulness: Mindfulness involves paying attention to the present moment without judgment. It can help you become more aware of your emotions as they arise, without reacting to them impulsively. Mindfulness techniques such as deep breathing, body scans, and meditation can help you manage and regulate your emotions effectively.

Emotional expression: Expressing your emotions in healthy ways can help you process and manage them. This can involve talking to a trusted friend or family member, writing in a journal, or engaging in creative outlets such as art, music, or dance. Finding healthy ways to express your emotions can prevent them from becoming bottled up and potentially leading to negative coping mechanisms such as substance abuse or emotional outbursts.

Cognitive restructuring: This involves identifying and challenging negative thought patterns that contribute to unhealthy emotional responses. By recognizing and changing negative thoughts, you can develop more adaptive ways of coping with difficult emotions. Techniques such as cognitive reframing, thought stopping, and cognitive-behavioral therapy (CBT) can be effective in helping you develop healthy coping mechanisms for managing emotions.

Self-care: Taking care of your physical, mental, and emotional well-being through self-care practices can help you build resilience and cope with emotions in a healthy way. This can involve getting enough sleep, eating a balanced diet, engaging in regular exercise, practicing relaxation techniques, and engaging in activities that you enjoy and find fulfilling.

Social support: Having a support system of trusted friends, family, or a therapist can provide you with a safe space to share your emotions and seek guidance. Talking to others can help you gain perspective, receive validation, and get practical advice on how to manage difficult emotions.

Problem-solving: Taking a proactive approach to addressing the underlying issues that are causing emotional distress can be a healthy coping mechanism. Identifying the problem, brainstorming potential solutions, and taking action can give you a sense of control and empower you to manage your emotions more effectively.

Time management: Poor time management can lead to stress and overwhelm, which can trigger emotional distress. Learning effective time management skills, setting realistic goals, and prioritizing tasks can help you manage your time more efficiently and reduce stress, allowing you to better cope with your emotions.

Remember, developing healthy coping mechanisms takes time and practice. It's important to be patient with yourself and seek support from a mental health professional if needed. Everyone's journey is different, and finding the coping mechanisms that work best for you may require some trial and error. But with practice and consistency, you can develop healthy coping mechanisms that help you manage your emotions in a positive and constructive way.

Chapter 8: Pursuing Your Passions and Goals

Identifying and nurturing personal strengths and interests

Identifying and nurturing personal strengths and interests is an important process for personal growth and self-improvement. Understanding what you are good at and what you are passionate about can help you make informed decisions about your career, hobbies, and personal development goals. Here are some steps you can take to identify and nurture your personal strengths and interests:

Reflect on your experiences: Take some time to reflect on your past experiences, both positive and negative, and think about what you enjoyed doing, what you were good at, and what gave you a sense of accomplishment. This could be anything from academic achievements, work projects, volunteer work, or personal hobbies. Identify patterns and common themes in your experiences to gain insights into your strengths and interests.

Assess your skills: Consider your skills and abilities, such as communication, leadership, problem-solving, creativity, and organization. Reflect on what comes naturally to you and what you excel at. Ask for feedback from others, such as friends, family, and colleagues, to gain additional insights into your strengths.

Follow your passions: Think about what you are truly passionate about and what genuinely interests you. It could be a particular subject, activity, or cause. When you are passionate about something, you are more likely to invest time and effort into it and excel in that area.

Experiment with new activities: Be open to trying new things and experimenting with different activities. This could include taking up a new hobby, joining a club or group, or volunteering for a cause that interests you. Trying new things can help you discover new strengths and interests that you may not have been aware of before.

Set goals and seek challenges: Set specific goals that align with your strengths and interests and push yourself to seek challenges that allow you to develop and showcase your skills. This could be taking on a new project at work, enrolling in a course or workshop, or participating in a competition or event related to your interests. Challenging yourself can help you grow and build confidence in your strengths.

Reflect on your values: Consider your values and beliefs, as they play an important role in shaping your interests and strengths. Reflect on what is truly important to you and how your strengths and interests align with your values. When your strengths and interests are aligned with your values, you are more likely to feel fulfilled and motivated.

Seek feedback and learn from failures: Be open to receiving feedback from others and learning from failures. Feedback can provide valuable insights into your strengths and areas for improvement. Embrace failures as learning opportunities and use them to reflect on what you could have done differently and how you can grow from them.

Remember, identifying and nurturing personal strengths and interests is a continuous process that requires self-reflection, self-awareness, and an open mindset. It may take time and effort, but investing in your strengths and interests can lead to personal growth, fulfillment, and success in various aspects of your life.

Setting and achieving realistic goals

Setting and achieving realistic goals is an important skill that can help you accomplish what you want in various aspects of your life, whether it's personal, professional, or academic. Here are some steps to help you set and achieve realistic goals:

Define your goal: Start by clearly defining what you want to achieve. Make sure your goal is specific, measurable, attainable, relevant, and time-bound (SMART). For example, instead of setting a vague goal like "I want to exercise more," set a SMART goal like "I want to exercise for 30 minutes, five days a week, for the next three months."

Break it down: Once you have a clear goal in mind, break it down into smaller, manageable steps. This will make it easier to work towards your goal and track your progress along the way. Create a timeline or a to-do list with deadlines for each step to keep yourself accountable.

Assess your resources: Consider what resources you have available to help you achieve your goal. This includes your time, skills, knowledge, and support system. Be realistic about what you can realistically accomplish given your current resources.

Set realistic expectations: It's important to set realistic expectations for yourself. Be honest about what you can realistically achieve given your current circumstances, and avoid setting overly ambitious goals that may be unattainable. Setting goals that are too difficult can lead to frustration and discouragement.

Develop an action plan: Create a detailed action plan that outlines the specific steps you need to take to achieve your goal. Be specific about what actions you will take, when you will take them, and how you will measure your progress. Break your goal down into smaller milestones, and celebrate your achievements along the way.

Stay motivated: Maintaining motivation is key to achieving your goals. Find ways to stay motivated, such as visualizing your success, reminding yourself of the benefits of achieving your goal, and seeking support from friends, family, or mentors. Keep yourself accountable by regularly reviewing your progress and adjusting your action plan as needed.

Be flexible: It's important to be flexible and adaptable as you work towards your goal. Life is unpredictable, and circumstances may change along the way. Be prepared to adjust your action plan as needed and reassess your goals if necessary. Don't be afraid to make changes and learn from any setbacks you encounter.

Celebrate your achievements: Finally, remember to celebrate your achievements along the way, no matter how small they may seem. Recognize your progress and reward yourself for your hard work and dedication. Celebrating your achievements will help you stay motivated and continue working towards your goal.

By following these steps and maintaining a positive and realistic mindset, you can set and achieve your goals in a more effective and sustainable way. Remember to be patient with yourself and stay committed to the process, and you will increase your chances of success.

Overcoming obstacles and setbacks

Overcoming obstacles and setbacks is an important skill that can help you navigate challenges and achieve your goals. Here are some tips on how to effectively overcome obstacles and setbacks:

Embrace a positive mindset: Maintaining a positive mindset can help you approach obstacles and setbacks with a proactive attitude. Rather than dwelling on the negative aspects of the situation, focus on what you can do to overcome the challenge and find solutions.

Set realistic expectations: It's important to set realistic expectations when facing obstacles and setbacks. Understand that challenges are a part of life, and setbacks are temporary setbacks. Set realistic goals and timelines for overcoming the obstacle, and be prepared for the possibility of setbacks along the way.

Learn from failures: Instead of viewing failures as defeats, see them as opportunities for growth and learning. Reflect on what went wrong, identify areas for improvement, and use the experience as a stepping stone towards future success.

Seek support: Don't be afraid to seek support from others when facing obstacles and setbacks. Talk to friends, family, mentors, or colleagues for advice, encouragement, or assistance. Having a support system can provide valuable insights, alternative perspectives, and emotional support during challenging times.

Develop a plan: Create a plan of action to overcome the obstacle or setback. Break the challenge down into smaller, manageable steps, and develop a strategy to tackle each step. Having a plan can help you stay focused, organized, and motivated as you work towards overcoming the obstacle.

Stay persistent and resilient: Overcoming obstacles and setbacks often requires persistence and resilience. Don't give up easily, and be prepared to face setbacks along the way. Stay committed to your goal, and keep pushing forward despite the challenges.

Take care of yourself: It's essential to take care of yourself physically, mentally, and emotionally when facing obstacles and setbacks. Make sure to get enough rest, eat healthy, exercise, and practice self-care. Taking care of yourself can help you stay physically and mentally strong, which can better equip you to overcome challenges.

Stay adaptable: Be open to adapting your approach if needed. Sometimes, obstacles and setbacks may require you to change your plans, be flexible, and try different strategies. Being adaptable can help you find new solutions and overcome challenges more effectively.

Remember, overcoming obstacles and setbacks takes time, effort, and perseverance. By maintaining a positive mindset, setting realistic expectations, learning from failures, seeking support, developing a plan, staying persistent and resilient, taking care of yourself, and staying adaptable, you can effectively overcome obstacles and setbacks and achieve your goals.

Fostering a growth mindset for success

Fostering a growth mindset is essential for achieving success in various aspects of life, including personal development, career growth, and lifelong learning. A growth mindset is the belief that intelligence, abilities, and skills can be developed through effort, perseverance, and learning from failures. It is in contrast to a fixed mindset, which assumes that abilities are fixed traits that cannot be changed.

Here are some ways to foster a growth mindset for success:

Embrace challenges: Challenges provide opportunities for growth and learning. Embrace challenges as a chance to learn and develop new skills, rather than avoiding them out of fear of failure. Embracing challenges with a positive attitude and a willingness to learn from them can lead to personal and professional growth.

Cultivate a love for learning: Embrace a lifelong learning mindset. Be curious and open to new ideas, experiences, and knowledge. Continuously seek opportunities to learn and expand your skills, whether it's through formal education, self-directed learning, or experiential learning.

Develop resilience: Failure and setbacks are part of the learning process. View them as opportunities to learn and improve, rather than as reasons to give up. Cultivate resilience by developing the ability to bounce back from failures, learn from them, and persevere despite obstacles.

Cultivate a positive attitude: Adopt a positive attitude towards yourself and your abilities. Believe in your potential to grow and improve. Replace negative self-talk and limiting beliefs with positive and empowering thoughts. Surround yourself with people who support and encourage your growth mindset.

Emphasize effort over outcome: Focus on the process and effort you put into a task or goal, rather than solely on the outcome. Recognize that effort and hard work are essential for growth and improvement. Acknowledge and celebrate your progress, regardless of the outcome.

Embrace feedback: Feedback, whether it's from mentors, peers, or supervisors, is invaluable for growth. Embrace feedback as an opportunity to learn and improve, rather than taking it as criticism. Be open to receiving feedback, and actively seek it out to gain insights into areas where you can grow and develop.

Set realistic goals: Set challenging but realistic goals that stretch your capabilities. Break down your goals into smaller, manageable steps, and celebrate your progress along the way. Adjust your goals as needed and be flexible in your approach, but stay committed to continuous improvement.

Practice self-reflection: Regularly reflect on your thoughts, behaviors, and actions to identify areas where you can improve. Be honest with yourself and take accountability for your mistakes and shortcomings. Learn from your experiences and use them as opportunities for growth.

In conclusion, fostering a growth mindset involves embracing challenges, cultivating a love for learning, developing resilience, maintaining a positive attitude, emphasizing effort over outcome, embracing feedback, setting realistic goals, and practicing self-reflection. By cultivating a growth mindset, you can unlock your potential for success and achieve your personal and professional goals.

Chapter 9: Practicing Mindfulness and Self-Reflection

Understanding the benefits of mindfulness for teens with ADHD

Mindfulness, which involves paying attention to the present moment with nonjudgmental awareness, can offer several benefits for teens with ADHD (Attention-Deficit/Hyperactivity Disorder). Here are some of the potential benefits of mindfulness for teens with ADHD:

Improved Focus and Attention: Mindfulness practices can help teens with ADHD enhance their ability to focus and sustain attention. Through mindfulness exercises, teens learn to be present in the moment without getting carried away by distractions, which can be particularly beneficial for managing ADHD symptoms related to inattention.

Increased Self-Awareness: Mindfulness encourages self-reflection and self-awareness, which can help teens with ADHD develop a deeper understanding of their thoughts, emotions, and behaviors. By becoming more aware of their internal experiences, teens can learn to recognize triggers, manage impulsive behaviors, and make more intentional choices.

Enhanced Emotional Regulation: Many teens with ADHD struggle with emotional regulation and may experience mood swings or impulsivity. Mindfulness can help teens develop emotional awareness and regulation skills by teaching them to observe their emotions without reacting to them impulsively. This can lead to better emotional self-regulation and reduced impulsivity.

Reduced Stress and Anxiety: Mindfulness practices have been shown to reduce stress and anxiety in various populations, including teens with ADHD. By learning to focus on the present moment and cultivate a nonjudgmental attitude, teens can reduce their stress levels and develop effective coping strategies for managing anxiety, which is often comorbid with ADHD.

Improved Executive Functioning Skills: Executive functioning skills, such as planning, organizing, and time management, are often impaired in individuals with ADHD. Mindfulness practices can help teens improve these skills by increasing their self-awareness, impulse control, and cognitive flexibility, which are essential for effective executive functioning.

Better Sleep: Many teens with ADHD struggle with sleep difficulties. Mindfulness can help teens relax and calm their minds, which can promote better sleep hygiene and improve the quality of their sleep.

Enhanced Interpersonal Skills: Mindfulness practices can also improve teens' interpersonal skills by teaching them to be present and fully engaged in social interactions without judgment. This can lead to better communication, empathy, and social connections, which are important for healthy relationships.

It's important to note that mindfulness is not a standalone treatment for ADHD, and it should be used as part of a comprehensive treatment plan that may include medication, therapy, and other strategies. However, incorporating mindfulness practices into the daily routine of teens with ADHD may offer additional benefits for managing their symptoms and improving their overall well-being. It's recommended to work with a qualified healthcare professional or mindfulness instructor to implement mindfulness practices tailored to the individual needs of teens with ADHD.

Practicing mindfulness exercises for focus and relaxation

Mindfulness exercises are a great way to cultivate focus and relaxation. Here are a few simple mindfulness exercises that you can practice:

Mindful Breathing: Find a quiet place to sit comfortably. Close your eyes and bring your attention to your breath. Notice the sensation of the breath as it enters and leaves your body. Don't try to change your breath in any way, just observe it as it is. If your mind wanders, gently bring your focus back to your breath. Practice this for a few minutes, gradually extending the duration of your practice over time.

Body Scan: Lie down or sit comfortably with your eyes closed. Start by bringing your attention to your toes and slowly move your attention up through your body, noticing any sensations, tension, or areas of relaxation. Pay attention to each part of your body as you scan from head to toe or vice versa. This can help you become more aware of your body and release any tension or stress.

Mindful Eating: Choose a small piece of food, such as a raisin or a piece of chocolate. Hold it in your hand and examine it closely, noticing its texture, color, and shape. Then bring it to your mouth and take a small bite, paying attention to the taste, texture, and sensation of chewing. Eat slowly and savor each bite, fully engaging your senses in the experience of eating.

Five Senses Check-In: Pause for a moment and bring your attention to your five senses - sight, hearing, taste, smell, and touch.

Notice what you can see around you, what you can hear, any tastes or smells in the air, and how your body feels as it touches surfaces. Take a few minutes to fully engage your senses and bring your focus to the present moment.

Mindful Walking: Find a quiet place to go for a walk, preferably in nature. As you walk, pay attention to each step, the sensation of your feet hitting the ground, the movement of your muscles, and the rhythm of your breath. Notice the sights, sounds, and smells around you without judgment, simply observing and being fully present in the act of walking.

Remember, mindfulness is about being fully present in the moment without judgment. It's normal for your mind to wander during these exercises, and when it does, gently bring your focus back to the exercise. With regular practice, mindfulness can help improve your focus and relaxation in various aspects of your life.

Reflecting on thoughts, emotions, and behaviors

Reflecting on our thoughts, emotions, and behaviors can be a valuable exercise for self-awareness and personal growth. By taking the time to examine these aspects of ourselves, we can gain insight into our patterns and habits, and better understand how they impact our lives.

When reflecting on our thoughts, it can be helpful to ask ourselves questions like, "What am I thinking about right now?" or "What assumptions or beliefs am I holding onto?" By identifying our thoughts, we can start to challenge any negative or unhelpful thinking patterns and replace them with more positive and constructive thoughts.

In terms of emotions, reflecting on how we feel in different situations can help us become more aware of our emotional responses and triggers. We can ask ourselves questions like, "What emotions am I feeling right now?" or "What situations or people tend to trigger certain emotions for me?" By understanding our emotions better, we can learn to regulate them more effectively and respond in healthier ways.

Finally, reflecting on our behaviors can help us identify areas where we may want to make changes or improvements. We can ask ourselves questions like, "What actions am I taking that are helping me achieve my goals?" or "What behaviors are holding me back?" By examining our behaviors, we can make more intentional choices about how we want to act and the kind of person we want to be.

Overall, reflecting on our thoughts, emotions, and behaviors can be a powerful tool for personal growth and self-awareness. By taking the time to examine these aspects of ourselves, we can develop a deeper understanding of who we are and how we can live more fulfilling and satisfying lives.

Cultivating self-awareness and self-compassion

Cultivating self-awareness and self-compassion are important skills that can help you lead a happier, more fulfilling life. Here are some tips on how to develop these skills:

Practice mindfulness: Mindfulness is the practice of being present in the moment without judgment. It can help you become more aware of your thoughts and feelings, and develop a more compassionate attitude towards yourself.

Journaling: Writing down your thoughts and feelings in a journal can help you gain clarity and insight into your emotions. This can help you develop a better understanding of yourself and your patterns of behavior.

Seek feedback: Ask trusted friends, family members, or a therapist for feedback on your behavior and how you come across to others. This can help you gain a more accurate understanding of yourself and how you're perceived by others.

Practice self-compassion: Instead of being critical of yourself, try to treat yourself with kindness and understanding. Remember that everyone makes mistakes, and that it's okay to be imperfect.

Take care of yourself: Make time for self-care activities such as exercise, meditation, or hobbies that bring you joy. Taking care of your physical and emotional needs can help you feel more centered and grounded.

Remember that cultivating self-awareness and self-compassion is an ongoing process. It takes time and effort to develop these skills, but the rewards are worth it. With practice, you can develop a deeper understanding of yourself and learn to treat yourself with kindness and compassion.

Chapter 10: Creating a Balanced Life

Balancing responsibilities, self-care, and leisure activities

Balancing responsibilities, self-care, and leisure activities can be a challenging task, but it's essential to maintain a healthy and fulfilling life. Here are some tips that can help you achieve balance in your daily routine:

Create a schedule: One of the best ways to ensure that you balance your responsibilities, self-care, and leisure activities is by creating a schedule. Identify the tasks you need to complete, allocate time for self-care and leisure activities, and stick to the schedule as much as possible.

Prioritize self-care: Self-care is crucial for your mental and physical well-being. Make sure you prioritize self-care activities such as exercise, meditation, and getting enough rest.

Delegate responsibilities: It's essential to delegate responsibilities to others to avoid feeling overwhelmed. Identify tasks that you can delegate to others and delegate them accordingly.

Learn to say no: It's okay to say no to commitments that may interfere with your self-care or leisure activities. Learn to prioritize your needs and say no when necessary.

Plan leisure activities: Plan leisure activities that you enjoy, and make time for them regularly. These activities can be a great way to recharge and reduce stress.

Be flexible: While having a schedule is important, it's also important to be flexible. Unexpected things can happen, and you may need to adjust your schedule accordingly.

Remember, balancing responsibilities, self-care, and leisure activities is an ongoing process. It's essential to be patient with yourself, and don't be afraid to make adjustments when necessary.

Developing healthy lifestyle habits, including sleep and exercise

Developing healthy lifestyle habits, including sleep and exercise, is crucial for maintaining physical and mental well-being. Here are some tips to help you get started:

Make a schedule: Set aside specific times for exercise and sleep. Try to stick to the same schedule every day, even on weekends.

Exercise regularly: Aim for at least 30 minutes of moderate exercise each day. This can include walking, jogging, cycling, or any other physical activity that you enjoy.

Prioritize sleep: Try to get 7-9 hours of sleep each night. Develop a bedtime routine that helps you relax and wind down before sleep, such as reading a book or taking a warm bath.

Eat a balanced diet: Make sure to eat a variety of nutrient-dense foods, including fruits, vegetables, whole grains, lean proteins, and healthy fats.

Stay hydrated: Drink plenty of water throughout the day to help your body function properly.

Manage stress: Find healthy ways to manage stress, such as meditation, deep breathing, or yoga.

Limit alcohol and caffeine: Too much alcohol or caffeine can disrupt sleep and lead to other health problems, so try to limit your intake.

Remember, developing healthy lifestyle habits takes time and effort, but the benefits are well worth it. Start small and make gradual changes to your routine, and soon you'll be on your way to a healthier, happier life.

Managing screen time and digital distractions

Managing screen time and digital distractions can be a challenge, especially in today's world where we rely heavily on technology for work, communication, entertainment, and more. Here are some tips to help you manage your screen time and avoid digital distractions:

Set boundaries: Create a schedule or routine for when you use technology and stick to it. For example, set aside specific times of the day for checking emails or social media, and avoid using technology during certain times, such as meal times or before bed.

Use apps or tools: There are several apps and tools available that can help you manage your screen time and minimize digital distractions. Some of these tools allow you to set limits on the amount of time you spend on certain apps or websites, while others can block notifications during certain times of the day.

Take breaks: Take regular breaks from technology to give your eyes and mind a rest. Get up and move around, take a walk outside, or do something else that doesn't involve technology.

Limit notifications: Turn off notifications for apps that are not essential, or limit them to only the most important ones. This can help reduce the temptation to check your phone or computer every time you receive a notification.

Practice mindfulness: Be mindful of your technology use and how it affects your mood, productivity, and overall well-being. Pay attention to how much time you spend on technology, and make adjustments as needed to ensure a healthy balance.

Remember, managing screen time and digital distractions is all about finding a healthy balance that works for you. By setting boundaries, using tools, taking breaks, limiting notifications, and practicing mindfulness, you can minimize the negative effects of technology and enjoy all the benefits it has to offer.

Cultivating a sense of balance and well-being in daily life

Cultivating a sense of balance and well-being in daily life is crucial for maintaining good mental and physical health. Here are some strategies that can help you achieve this:

Develop a daily routine: Establishing a routine can help you feel more in control of your life and reduce stress. Plan your day ahead of time, schedule your tasks, and prioritize what's important.

Get enough sleep: Getting enough sleep is crucial for maintaining good mental and physical health. Aim for 7-8 hours of sleep per night and try to stick to a consistent sleep schedule.

Practice mindfulness: Mindfulness is the practice of being fully present and engaged in the moment. Try to incorporate mindfulness into your daily routine by taking a few minutes each day to focus on your breath, notice your surroundings, and tune into your body.

Stay physically active: Exercise has numerous benefits for physical and mental health. Find an activity you enjoy and make it a regular part of your routine.

Eat a healthy diet: Eating a balanced diet that includes plenty of fruits, vegetables, whole grains, and lean protein can help you feel energized and improve your overall well-being.

Connect with others: Social connections are important for maintaining good mental health. Make time to connect with friends, family, or other people who share your interests.

Manage stress: Stress is a natural part of life, but chronic stress can have negative effects on your health. Find healthy ways to manage stress, such as meditation, deep breathing exercises, or taking a walk in nature.

By incorporating these strategies into your daily routine, you can cultivate a sense of balance and well-being in your life. Remember, it's important to take care of yourself in order to live your best life.

Epilogue: Embracing Your Potential

Reflecting on the journey of self-care with ADHD

Self-care is crucial for everyone, but it can be especially challenging for individuals with ADHD. The journey of self-care with ADHD is often a rocky one, filled with obstacles, setbacks, and moments of triumph.

One of the most important aspects of self-care for individuals with ADHD is understanding the unique challenges that come with the condition. ADHD can make it difficult to focus, regulate emotions, and manage time effectively. As a result, individuals with ADHD may struggle with basic self-care tasks such as maintaining a healthy sleep schedule, exercising regularly, and eating nutritious meals.

To overcome these challenges, individuals with ADHD may need to develop a personalized self-care plan that takes into account their unique needs and abilities. This may involve seeking support from mental health professionals, creating a structured routine, practicing mindfulness, and incorporating strategies such as exercise, meditation, and cognitive-behavioral therapy.

Another important aspect of self-care with ADHD is learning to manage stress and anxiety effectively. Individuals with ADHD are often prone to experiencing high levels of stress and anxiety, which can exacerbate symptoms and make it even more challenging to maintain good self-care habits. Mindfulness practices, such as meditation and deep breathing, can be helpful for managing stress and anxiety, as can regular exercise and engaging in enjoyable activities.

Finally, it's important to recognize that the journey of self-care with ADHD is an ongoing process that requires patience, perseverance, and self-compassion. There will be setbacks and challenges along the way, but with the right tools and support, it's possible to develop effective self-care habits that can improve overall well-being and quality of life.

Celebrating progress and achievements

Celebrating progress and achievements is an important aspect of life that helps us recognize and appreciate our efforts and hard work. It also serves as a motivator to keep pushing ourselves towards further progress and success. Here are some tips on how to celebrate progress and achievements:

Acknowledge the accomplishment: Take a moment to acknowledge and appreciate the progress you have made or the achievement you have accomplished. This can be done by simply taking a moment to reflect on what you have achieved and what it means to you.

Share the news: Share the news with family and friends who have been supportive throughout the process. Let them know how much their encouragement and support has meant to you.

Treat yourself: Celebrate by treating yourself to something you have been wanting or have been putting off. This could be a nice dinner, a weekend getaway, or a new piece of clothing or gadget.

Thank those who helped: Take the time to thank those who have helped you along the way. This could be a mentor, a coach, a teacher, or anyone who has played a supportive role in your journey.

Plan for the next steps: Celebrating progress and achievements is also a great time to plan for the next steps in your journey. Use this momentum to set new goals and keep pushing forward.

Remember, celebrating progress and achievements is not just about the end result, but also about recognizing the effort and hard work that went into achieving it. So take the time to celebrate and enjoy the moment!

Embracing your unique strengths and talents

Embracing your unique strengths and talents is a powerful way to increase your confidence, motivation, and happiness in life. When you understand your strengths and focus on using them, you can achieve more and feel more fulfilled in your personal and professional life.

Here are some tips for embracing your unique strengths and talents:

Identify your strengths: Start by taking some time to reflect on your past experiences, successes, and challenges. What are the skills, qualities, and traits that helped you succeed? You can also ask friends, family, and colleagues for feedback on what they think your strengths are.

Celebrate your strengths: Once you have identified your strengths, celebrate them and recognize their value. Instead of focusing on your weaknesses, focus on what you are good at and find ways to use your strengths to your advantage.

Develop your strengths: Once you know your strengths, you can focus on developing them further. Take courses, read books, or seek out mentors who can help you develop your skills and knowledge.

Find opportunities to use your strengths: Look for opportunities in your personal and professional life to use your strengths. If you are a great communicator, for example, look for opportunities to speak in public or lead a team meeting.

Embrace your uniqueness: Remember that everyone has different strengths and talents, and that's what makes us unique. Embrace your individuality and don't be afraid to let your true self shine through.

By embracing your unique strengths and talents, you can increase your self-awareness, confidence, and motivation. So take the time to identify your strengths, celebrate them, develop them, and find opportunities to use them in your life.

Looking towards a bright future with confidence and resilience.

Looking towards a bright future with confidence and resilience can be challenging at times, especially when facing obstacles or setbacks. However, with the right mindset and approach, it is possible to cultivate a positive outlook and the ability to bounce back from difficulties.

One important aspect of building confidence and resilience is to focus on your strengths and accomplishments. Take some time to reflect on your past successes and the skills and qualities that helped you achieve them. Use these as a foundation to build upon and remind yourself of your abilities and potential.

Another key factor is to adopt a growth mindset. Embrace challenges as opportunities for growth and learning, rather than viewing them as insurmountable obstacles. Recognize that setbacks and failures are a natural part of the learning process, and use them as opportunities to adjust your approach and try again.

It can also be helpful to cultivate a support system of people who encourage and uplift you. Surround yourself with positive influences and seek out mentors or role models who embody the qualities you aspire to.

Finally, practice self-care and prioritize your physical and emotional wellbeing. Engage in activities that bring you joy and relaxation, such as exercise, meditation, or spending time with loved ones. By taking care of yourself, you will be better equipped to handle challenges and face the future with confidence and resilience.

www.ingramcontent.com/pod-product-compliance
Lightning Source LLC
Chambersburg PA
CBHW070834250726
48662CB00003B/1226